The Night That Changed a Life

(The Unspoken After Labour)

Cassandra Robertson

The Night That Changed a Life
Copyright © 2023 by Cassandra Robertson
All Rights Reserved

No part of this book may be reproduced or transmitted in any form or by any means, electronic or mechanical, including photocopying, recording, or by any information storage and retrieval system without the written permission of the author, except where permitted by law.

I dedicate this book to all the women and men out there who have become single parents and show their loyalty to their children. I would also like to dedicate this to all the young ladies who think that having a child is a walk in the park with no complications to come along with it.

Acknowledgements

Girls think that having a baby is a walk in the park, but the untold story of labour and delivery is that anything can come out of having a baby just like Emerald ended up having in the story. Further, when starting out dating someone, they may show you how nice and respectful they are at first, but this is only when they have just met you. Later, in the relationship, they often show their true colors so always keep your eyes open to behaviour changes.

Table of Contents

Chapter One 1

Chapter Two 5

Chapter Three 9

Chapter Four 14

Chapter Five 19

Chapter Six 22

Chapter Seven 25

Chapter Eight 28

About the Author 33

Chapter One

Once upon a time on a cold wet day, in mid-February at 1:00pm, Mother Crystal had to work both her jobs out of town. Daughter Emerald had an appointment with a breastfeeding counsellor. She was suffering from hot and cold chills during the day, she was extremely tired. Emerald's older brother Edward used Alex's car to drive Emerald, Frank, and Sapphire to the breastfeeding clinic appointment. On their way to the appointment, Emerald asked, "Is anyone else feeling cold?" Frank replied, "No, you are crazy!"

Emerald ignored Frank's comment as she was not wanting to fight in front of baby Sapphire. Edward let Emerald know, "We are just a block away from the clinic then hopefully you will be warmer inside the building, let me know when you are done with your appointment."

At 3:00pm, Emerald pulled into the clinic's driveway. She got the baby car seat out of the car, but with how weak she was already, Emerald requested Frank, "Can you carry the baby to the office? I am feeling so weak that I am afraid I will drop her."

Frank replied, "Stop being so much of a wimp. You are her mother." Emerald picked up the car seat with the baby inside of it. She knew it was going to take a while to get to the doors. Frank and Emerald finally arrived at the doors of the clinic just on time, as Emerald had to go extra slow since she was carrying Sapphire while she was weak.

While at the appointment, Emerald was learning how to latch baby Sapphire the different ways. She was having a challenging time as she was shaking quite a bit. Emerald was trying her best not to show how cold and discomfort she was while in the appointment. Emerald had 30 more minutes until her appointment was over when the counsellor noticed Emerald shaking. She asked Emerald, "Are you cold?" Emerald replied, "No, I'm not." The counsellor asked, "Could I have a brief moment without your daughter?" Emerald agreed to talk briefly without her baby in the room. After the session, another counsellor took baby Sapphire while Emerald went to another room with her counsellor.

During the talk, Emerald told the counsellor, "I have been feeling very off all day." The counsellor replied, "Can you please explain to me how long before this morning did this off feeling happen?" Emerald hesitantly answered, "This morning at around 8:00am, I woke, and my pajamas were all wet from me sweating in my sleep!"

During Emerald's talk, her boyfriend Frank was being impatient while sitting with the other counsellor and baby Sapphire. Frank stated to the counsellor holding Sapphire, "Can I have the baby?"

The counsellor replied, "Emerald asked if I could hang onto her while those two talked." Not happy with the reply, Frank started to raise his voice, "Give me my F**king baby now!" The other counsellor hesitantly just stared at Frank before replying, "I will wait until Emerald and my colleague come back from the other room. Thank you."

After over 20 minutes, Emerald and the counsellor came back to the room with Frank, Sapphire, and her colleague. Before they were able to say a word about the next appointment, Frank started yelling at Emerald, "Why do you have to always whine about the smallest things?"

Emerald did not know how to answer his hostile question; she asked for baby Sapphire, got her ready to head home. Frank still angry, asked, "Why the hell did you not just let me hang onto Sapphire?" Emerald replied, "I was not chancing that you would strand me while I am struggling with this transition in life." The counsellors could see that Emerald was struggling with putting Sapphire into her car seat. Frank was getting more impatient waiting for the baby to be done up, as Emerald could only go so fast because of how weak she was.

At that time, Frank started arguing with both counsellors and Emerald. "If you two would get off your ass and assist her, then the baby would be already done up, and we would be already out of your guy's damn clinic." The counsellors looked at each other, then looked at Emerald with a puzzled look on their faces questioning whether they should allow her and baby Sapphire to leave with Frank. The first counsellor asked, "Emerald, are you going to feel safe going home with him and the baby?"

Also asked, "Are you guys going to be alone?" Emerald replied to both, "I feel safe to leave with him. He will calm down." Emerald also explained, "No my brother Edward is picking up three up." Once the counsellors knew that Emerald and Sapphire were going to be okay. They made sure that they got to the vehicle safely. They both told Emerald, "If you need any help with latching the baby more, do not hesitate to give us a call," along with "If you are needing medical assistance do not hesitate to call 911."

Chapter Two

While on their way home, Frank asked Emerald, "Why did they say if you need assistance, to not hesitate to call 911?" Emerald replied, "With the way I have been feeling all day, they think I could end up getting worse?"

Frank replied, "I do not think that you need help. You just need to learn to not argue so much!" Emerald asked, "Frank why do you always seem to blame me for everything when we both know you start with the fighting over getting mad at small things like this morning baby Sapphire waking up and you yelling at her."

Frank replied, "I was just tired, and Sapphire woke just when I was closing my eyes to sleep." That conversation went on until they got back home. Emerald asked her brother Edward, "Since Frank won't carry Sapphire, will you carry her into the house? I feel too weak?"

Edward replied, "Anything for my Favorite sister!"

While at home, Emerald called her mom to touch base on her appointment. While on the phone, Emerald filled her mom in on the appointment and events that followed. "Hello, Mom, I have not been feeling very well. At the appointment, I was having a hard time with latching Sapphire." Crystal asked, "Why, what happened"? Emerald, shivering, replied, "I have been too shaky all day." With this information, Crystal asked, "Emerald, do you think you need to go see a doctor, or can you wait until I get home?" Emerald replied, "I think I can wait until you are home unless things get worse." Crystal said, "Emerald, you soak in a warm bath to help you feel better, then go I am off work at 11:00pm, Edward can drive you to get looked at." Emerald agreed to get a warm bath, while they hung up the phone, Emerald went slowly up the stairs. She got to the bathroom, where she started to run a tub with warm water. She got undressed and climbed into the warm tub by herself; she did not lock the bathroom door in case of an emergency. While in the tub, Emerald fell asleep, the warm water was relaxing her body. Emerald's tub water had turned very red fast, the red of the water was a bad sign!

While Emerald was in the tub, her brother Joe watched Sapphire and cared for her. Emerald woke up to the slamming of the door from Frank storming out of the house. Frank was pissed off from arguing with Joe about who was watching baby Sapphire. That was when she noticed the colour change of the bathtub water. Frank returned to the house, slamming every door he had entered. That time Emerald was feeling worse than earlier. She just wanted her mom. With Emerald being too weak to get out of the bathtub by herself, she started to panic. While Emerald was panicking, Frank went to the bathroom and informed Emerald, "You need to get out of that bathtub NOW." Emerald replied, "Frank, leave me alone. I do not want you to touch me; I only want my mom." Frank was very unhappy with her answer and replied, "Well, that cannot happen. She isn't even at the house." Frank then stated, "You need to get out; there is no other choice." Emerald just kept replying, "I want my mom, leave me alone Frank!" Frank would not leave her alone. He was just working the sick young mother up, which was not helping with her sickness.

While she was yelling for her mom, her brother Joe was sitting in the living room with baby Sapphire at the time of the arguing between Frank and Emerald. Joe decided it was time to get on the phone with their mom, Crystal, at work. He explained Emerald was not feeling well at all, as she was yelling for Crystal. While on the phone, Crystal could hear all the yelling coming from her house. Crystal asked Joe, "Is that Emerald that I can hear yelling"? Joe replied, "Yes, Mom she is just wanting you, no one else."

Crystal was hoping she would be okay till 11:00 when she would be home. Joe was not sure if Emerald could wait that long to get looked at. With the thought, Joe asked, "Mom, maybe you should call Dad and fill him in with what is happening at the house." Crystal replied, "I do not want to work your father up while he is in hospital recovering from pneumonia." Joe replied, "Yes, but if something bad happened to Emerald, Dad does not know. He will be more upset with everyone for not informing him." Crystal agreed to give the hospital where her husband Alex was. Joe and Crystal said 'goodbye' and hung up the phone.

Chapter Three

When Crystal was off the phone with Joe, she called the hospital where her husband Alex was. She wanted to speak to him. When Crystal called the hospital, she talked to a volunteer at the front desk. She asked, "Can you transfer me to the floor my husband Alex is on?"

The volunteer asked, "Please hold?" While on hold, Crystal waited 10 minutes until a nurse on Alex's floor answered the nursing phone. The nurse answered, "Hello, how may I assist you?" Crystal asked, "Is there any way that I can talk to my husband Alex?"

The nurse asked, "Can you give me a few minutes?"

Before Crystal could reply, the nurse already put her on hold. About 5 minutes went by until Crystal heard the nurse come back to the phone. The nurse informed Crystal, "You have about 10 minutes as I cannot keep this phone tied up too long as other patient's families call on it."

Crystal stated, "Hello Alex, is that you?" Even though Alex was just recovering replied, "Yes, Hunny, it is me. What is wrong?"

Crystal went on telling him, "Emerald is unwell at home and is refusing to get out of the tub." Alex replied, "How am I supposed to assist while I am at the hospital?" Crystal gave an idea, "Call the house and talk to Joe. He may be able to get her out she needs to be seen by a doctor." She told him what was going on; he was unwell in the hospital, so he could not get home. She also told him that Emerald would not get out of the bathtub for Frank, and she was calling for Crystal from the bathroom. Alex replied, "Let me call the house to try and talk with her about how important it is to get out of the tub!"

Crystal agreed with Alex and stated, "Okay, love you, Hunny!" Then, they both hung up the phone before Alex could call the house. Once off the telephone, he called his home. Alex spoke to Joe; he was informed that Emerald was worse. She was in the tub with absolutely no strength to get up. Alex said, "Help her get up and ready, get an ambulance to get her to the hospital." Joe replied, "What if she does not let me?" Alex replied, "Put me on speaker and go into the bathroom, I will talk to her." Joe answered, "Dad, you are not well enough to get her to listen. Let me try to get her out!" Alex replied, "I understand, Joe. If you need any more help, call 911." Joe and Alex said goodbye, and Joe put Sapphire in her swing to sleep and went upstairs.

While Joe was on his way up the stairs, he could tell Frank was making things worse. Joe told Frank, "Leave her alone and grab her clothes." Frank grabbed a towel, he tried to put it around Emerald, but she would not let him. Joe said, "Emerald's dad says to get out of the bathtub and get looked at." Emerald replied, "If he is the one helping me, then I am not moving. I do not feel safe with him lifting me out. I will fall in his care. Joe replied, "Emerald, will you let me assist you in getting out of the tub?" Emerald replied, "If it is only you, yes." Joe assisted Emerald with climbing out of the tub. He had to take all her weight as she could not stand on her own with how weak she is.

Emerald would only let Joe assist with getting her out, putting a towel around her, and assisting her to her room to get dress. She did not want Frank to touch her as he was only yelling and screamed, she felt as if she would fall because he would not like how she would assist with her weakness. They went to Emerald's room as it seemed as though Frank only got a towel. Joe assisted Emerald with Pajama Pants and a Sweater as it would help keep her warm. After getting dressed, Joe instructed Frank, "Call for the ambulance, please." Frank hesitantly called 911 for an ambulance. Frank was not the greatest at explaining what was going on, as he believed that Emerald was just trying to get attention. Dispatch for 911 answered, "Hello, do you need Fire, Police, or Ambulance?" Frank answered, "My wife's family says that she needs an ambulance." Dispatch replied, "I will transfer you."

When the ambulance Dispatch came on the phone, they asked, "What is the emergency?" Frank replied, "My in-laws believe that my wife needs to be seen by a doctor." Dispatch asked, "What is wrong with your wife?" Frank hesitantly replied, "She is shaking, bleeding badly. Just had a baby six days ago." Dispatch let Frank know, "We have an ambulance en route. Please have any clothes or medication that she needs to take ready to hand over." Frank answered, "I'm not sure why you guys are going to waste your time coming here, as it is normal for a new mother to bleed." Dispatch replied, "Sir, you are the one who called for the help. The ambulance will be there in 5 minutes. Call if anything gets worse. Goodbye."

The ambulance showed up at 6:00pm to find Emerald having trouble; the Paramedics took her blood pressure, it was reading a little higher than normal, Paramedics Gile instructed, "Emerald, you look in bad shape, I feel you should see a doctor". Emerald replied, stuttering with her words, "I want to, want to wait until my mom is home." Gile explained, "Emerald, if you don't go, know you may not survive until she is home!" Paramedic Gile inquired, "Joe, can you help me bring your sister to the ambulance?" Joe replied, "Let me get her left side!" Joe and Gile guided Emerald down the stairs and out the door to the ambulance. They put her on the stretcher. While Joe headed back into the house to be with Sapphire, the ambulance started to pull out of the driveway.

While en route to the hospital, Emerald drifted in and out of consciousness. Emerald had just Pajama pants and a sweater, no socks, underwear, or anything else needed. When Gile looked over at Emerald, he saw that she was in distress. He quickly turned from zone 2 to 3, lights flashing and sirens going until he hit the ambulance port doors. The ambulance was dispatched to the hospital to let them know they were 2 minutes out and had a code blue on board to be prepared with a room. The ambulance driver and co-worker Gile got the stretcher out of the ambulance and started their way into the hospital awaiting them with three nurses.

Chapter Four

Once she arrived at the hospital, she was taken right to acute care. Monitors got hooked up, a small examination was done. A nurse was assigned to her right after. With Emerald at the hospital, her brother Joe got on the phone to call their mother, Crystal. "Mom, Emerald has been brought by ambulance to the local hospital." With the shock of the news, Crystal hung up the phone before being able to say thank you and goodbye. Finding out that her daughter went to the hospital, Crystal called her boss and filled her in. Crystal asked her boss, "Is there any way I can leave early?" Her boss asked, "Is your daughter in that bad of shape?" Crystal explained, "My daughter is in the local hospital in worse shape than she was early." Crystal's boss replied, "Just wait until your co-worker arrives. I will call them right now.

Crystal and her boss hung up the phone so that her co-worker could get the call. With the permission to leave early, Crystal phoned home Joe picked up the phone. "Hello, Mom," Joe answered. Crystal replied, "Hello Joe, where is your brother Edward? Joe replied, "He just left to pick a friend up and drop them off. Why?" Crystal was unhappy with what she had just been told, so she asked

Joe, "When he gets home, get him to call me as soon as possible!"

An estimated 5 minutes went by, and Crystal's work phone rang. It was Crystal's house phone number.

"Hello," said Crystal. Edward being on the other side, "Hello, Mom. You wanted me to call you?" Crystal replied, "I need you to come pick me up with Dad's car, bring me to the hospital where your sister is."

Once her co-worker came in, her older son came to pick her up. Edward drove her to the emergency entrance where Crystal got out. While entering the emergency doors, Crystal's eyes were filled with tears from how scared she was for her daughter. Crystal approached the tri-ad nurse station to inquire about Emerald being there. "Hello," Crystal states, in reply, tri-ad stated, "How many I help you." Crystal answered, "I am looking for my daughter Emerald. Can you locate her?" Tri-ad replied, "Yes give me a second." The nurse ran her name, she was only about to confirm at that point yes she was the Emerald that Crystal was talking about. Tri-ad stated, "She is in the back, but no one can go back yet, so please have a seat, and someone will call you in."

Crystal was not allowed to enter to see her daughter. She waited the 5 minutes, then went back up to the nursing station. At that time, she asked 'what was happening.' The nurse behind the glass had no information on patients in the back, so said she, "I am sorry, but I could not answer any of your questions." While Crystal was waiting to go back to see her daughter, Frank showed up at the hospital. Frank being told the same information as Crystal frustrated Frank, so he decided to leave. Seemed like hours, but about 20 minutes later, the nurse from the acute care area came over. That nurse said, "Are you Emerald's mom? If so, can you please follow me to your daughter?" Crystal got up from the seat she was sitting on and followed the nurse.

Crystal followed threw two doors; while arriving at acute care, another nurse asked for Crystal to wait outside as she needed to examine Emerald again. The nurse informed Crystal, "It is only going to take another 5 minutes, then you can go into her cubicle. Crystal replied, "Okay, I will wait to be informed I am allowed in."

The nurse came out.

"Mom you can go in and see your daughter now. While walking into Emerald's cubicle, Crystal noticed all the monitors and wires that Emerald was hooked up to. All the numbers kept going up, and several beepings were coming from the monitor. While visiting Emerald, Crystal started to notice that Emerald's pulse was wrong. The number was too high, so she approached the nurse and spoke briefly. Crystal stated, "My daughter has a high pulse!" The nurse said, "Everything is okay." So, Crystal went back to the cubicle to visit with Emerald longer.

Emerald was very cold. Crystal went to the nurse station, the nurse came in, looked over, checked the monitors then asked Emerald if she was a little cold. Emerald replied, "I'm freezing." So, the nurse got her a warm sheet. Crystal asked, "Emerald, who is at home with the baby?" Emerald replied, "Mommy, *bobfer* Joe is watching Sapphire." That was when Crystal noticed that Emerald started to slur her words, not making sense when talking. Emerald was getting frustrated with people not understanding what she said.

The monitors kept beeping more. Crystal went to ask why the monitors kept beeping. The nurse came in, did a quick look, and said, "Everything is okay. They are beeping as it seems her numbers are a little high but come back down on their own." Crystal did not believe it because Emerald was getting paler and shaking badly. She was not keeping her body temperature when Crystal would feel her; she would be freezing to touch. At least an hour went by, Emerald was getting weaker, and her body was shaking worse. The nurse examined her at least ten times, she kept saying she was fine. Crystal was talking to Emerald; she was having trouble breathing. Crystal was looking at the monitor; she noticed that the pulse in the neck area was too fast. She left the cubicle one more time,

Emerald's nurse was not available. Crystal waved down a nurse at the nurse's station that seemed to be nice. She wanted to let them know that Emerald looked worse than she was before Crystal saw her.

Chapter Five

The nurse there listened to Crystal, she was saying, "I'll let her nurse know when she's back." Before Crystal got back to the cubicle, Emerald was screaming, "I cannot breathe, I cannot breathe, Mom, I need help, help me please!" Crystal attempted to enter the cubicle, but the nurse had entered. You could hear all the beeping. Once the nurse entered the cubicle, Emerald was shaking badly, gasping for air. The nurse called a code blue. Several nurses, and doctors entered the cubicle, and they pulled the curtain. No one was allowed to enter. As they started to all surround Emerald, she was still yelling for her mom to help her until she was unconscious.

No one would speak to Crystal who was alone, she could only stand and hear the commotion behind the curtains. She could hear the paddles being used, a doctor saying clear then another says push the button. There were four or five clears called out. Finally, a doctor said, "Okay, she is breathing, okay."

Crystal was still not allowed in her daughter's cubical, as it seemed though doctors were making sure that Emerald did not need any more assistance from the code blue team. Seemed like forever, at least a half hour passed with tears, worries, and thoughts like what is happening. Praying saying please help my twenty-year-old baby she must pull through; her daughter Sapphire needs her.

Another half hour went by before Crystal was allowed back to be by Emerald's side. Crystal noticed that oxygen and an IV was attached to Emerald. Her breathing was not normal, but she was deep breathing lots. Crystal asked, "How are you feeling now, Emerald?" Emerald had a tough time replying, but she stated, "The Oxygen is helping me breathe a little bit more than I was 10 minutes ago." Her nurse came in more frequently. Emerald was so tired that she dozed off more for over an hour before waking up after longer hours. During the next hour, a lab technician came in with orders to draw blood. The lab technician informed Emerald, "I am needing to take your blood. Doctors are looking to see if the infection has gotten into your blood." Crystal asked the technician, "What infection are the doctors looking at in Emerald's blood?"

The technician could not answer that question. All she could tell Crystal was she had to bring in two huge bottles and had to draw blood to fill them. Crystal asked, "Why so much blood?" All she could find out was for the next three hours. They would be back to fill at least two more bottles. Crystal asked the technician, "Does the doctor think that my daughter is going to be able to go home before tomorrow?" The lab technician could not answer that question and stated, "Maybe ask her nurse the next time they come in, as I only take the blood." Crystal asked the nurse when she came in, "What was the doctor looking for?" The nurse did not have an answer but stated, "When I have answers, I will let you know." The no response of any of her questions was getting Crystal frustrated. At least an hour later, the doctor came in to examine Emerald. Crystal asked in hopes for answers, "What infection are you hoping to locate from her blood?" The doctor explained, "We are hoping to find out that the infection that we think she has is not speeding to her blood."

Crystal asked more questions like, "What is wrong? Is she going to be okay?" All the doctors could tell Crystal was more blood work was needed, and, hopefully answers would come then. Around 1:00am, Emerald was more stable and relaxed. She woke a little longer. Emerald asked her mom if she checked on how Joe was doing with Sapphire, also how she was going to be fed. Emerald was asking, as she was concerned about her baby's nutarian as the last feed was hours ago. Crystal left Emeralds cubical so that she could set outside to use her cell phone to call home and see how things were.

Chapter Six

Crystal dialed her house phone number it rang "Hello Joe how is things going with Sapphire." Joe let Crystal know, "Sapphire was in amazing hands, even though he was unsure what he was doing with a newborn baby." Crystal asked, "Have you feed Sapphire, what did you get her to eat as she is not on solids being only six days old?" Joe said to his mom, "I went to shoppers and picked up some pre-made baby formula as well as a few steroid baby nipples." Crystal replied, "I am happy you could get help from the workers to get the right things for Sapphire." Crystal also assured him that she would be home in a little to retrieve Sapphire so he could go to bed. Crystal returned and told Emerald not to worry that Joe got some formula for Sapphire and was doing great with her. That put a smile on Emerald's face. She was very worried about her six-day-old daughter.

Frank finally returned to the hospital and made a big scene at the nurse's station. Demanded to see his wife. The nurse came back to speak to Emerald to confirm that he was her boyfriend and in a bad mood. Emerald stated, "You can let him back but please do not leave me alone with him." While Frank walked past the nursing station, the nurses informed each other to keep an eye on him as their patient seem to get a little stress just hearing he was here at the hospital. The nurse monitored his actions while in the cubicle. Crystal and Frank do not agree completely, Crystal walked over to the nurse station and asked, "Can you guys make sure that she is not left alone with him?" The nurses asked, "Where are you heading, and do you want us to call you if anything happens?" Crystal let the nurses know that she had a little bundle of joy to go take off a tired uncle's hands. Crystal called her older son Edward at the house, she inquired, "Edward anyway you can come pick me up where you dropped of me at the hospital?" Edward answered, "I will be on my way and be there soon." Crystal left just after 1:30am, she had Edward come pick her up. She went home and took over the grandma roll so Sapphire's uncle Joe could get some sleep.

While Frank was, still at the hospital until Emerald was able to be discharged. Then 6:00am came around, Emerald was doing better. She was released with orders to return at 9:00am for an ultrasound. She came home with Frank who was arguing about Emerald not sleeping upstairs with him. While entering the house, he got rough, grabbed Emerald's arm trying to force her to go upstairs. Crystal said, "Frank let go of Emerald's arm and go to bed. She needs to sleep as Sapphire will soon be awake for a feeding."

The Night That Changed a Life

Frank stomped up every step muddling to himself. Emerald curled up and crashed on the comfortable couch. Sapphire was asleep in her bassinet, which Uncle Joe brought down earlier that day. Everyone slept but it was a rough night. Sapphire woke before 7:00 am, Emerald fed her but was weak. While Emerald was finishing Sapphire feed, Crystal went upstairs to get clean clothes, socks, underwear, and a few pads for Emerald. She helped Emerald get dressed for her appointment at the hospital. She let Emerald know that at the appointment, she was a call away for when she found out any news of what was going to happen with her.

Chapter Seven

That day there was no work for Crystal so she could be there for Sapphire while Emerald went back to the hospital. Before 8:30 am, Emerald left with Frank, he was being a little rude. Frank and Emerald arrived at the ultrasound department, they took Emerald's information and asked her to wait in the waiting room for her name to be called. The ultrasound tech came out and said, "Is there an Emerald in the waiting room?" Emerald got up, "I am here." The ultrasound tech asked, "Please, follow me to the ultrasound room."

Emerald got her ultrasound done; she asked the tech "Where do I go to wait for the results?" The tech replied, "If you go to the emergency department, they will call you in when they have the results." Frank and Emerald walked over to the Emergency, they found out they had to get registered. Emerald went to tri-ad, "I just had an ultrasound done and was told to come here for my results." The tri-ad stated, "Please take a seat in this waiting room and someone will call you in." It took until after 10:30am for the doctors to call Emerald in once the ultrasound was done. A nurse from zone 5.

"Is there a person named Emerald here waiting?" Emerald answered, "I am here waiting yes." The nurse replied, "Please follow me to zone 5 and sit in room 034." Not long after Emerald and Frank went into room 034 the doctor came in, "Emerald I will be sending you to the second floor, you are needing to have surgery." Emerald and Frank went to the second floor and await surgery.

It turned out that there was still some afterbirth left in the womb. The reason Emerald was so sick was that poison was settling in, causing the fever, chills, and shakes. Emerald was about to call home and tell her mom everything.

Emerald: "Hello, mom I have some news for you, not the news we wanted to hear." Crystal "Please explain what has been found?"

Emerald: "The ultrasound showed that doctors left some afterbirth in me which has caused an infection all threw my body."

While on the phone, Crystal could hear Frank yelling at Emerald. He said, "When we get back to your parents, you are going upstairs."

Emerald said, "I am tired! Please stop!"

Crystal could not handle how Frank was treating her daughter while she was sick; she hung up the phone without saying goodbye to Emerald.

Emerald's surgent came out and asked, "Emerald are you here?"

Emerald answered, "Yes, I am here and waiting." He let Emerald know, "I will be back out in 5 minutes to get you." Emerald replied, "Alright I will be waiting." At 3:00pm, the surgent finally came out and stated, "Emerald, we are ready for you to come into the room. Frank you can wait in the waiting area if you would like."

Frank did not like that; he had to wait in the hospital and left the hospital. On return to the hospital Frank still was waiting as it was still only 04:30pm and she was not going to be out for another half an out or so. The doctor came out, "Frank are you waiting for Emerald?"

Frank replied, "Yes, can we go home know?"

The doctor said, "She has to go to the recovery room first." Frank not liking that answer he started yelling, "I AM BRING HER HOME KNOW."

The doctor replied, "Sorry that I can see you are upset with what I told you, but she is not ready yet." The doctor also let him know, "I am going to calling her mom at the house to touch base as Emerald asked me to."

Chapter Eight

Crystal had to wait until after 5:00pm for more news. A doctor called her to inform that surgery went well Emerald was in recovery would be about another hour. Also, he said, "The guy here is not understanding, he is very argumentative." Crystal asked, "Why is he upset; he is not the easiest to handle." The doctor explained, "He is yelling that he is bring your daughter home, even though she needs to go to the 6th floor." Crystal asked, "Can anyone come and visit her on the 6th floor when she gets there?" The doctor assured her, "Yes, anyone can come and see her when she is there." Crystal stated, "Thank you for calling me, and letting me know this goodbye." Once off the phone from the doctor she called the hospital to speak with Alex. His nurse reassured her that he was doing well. She also let Crystal know that he had concerns about their daughter.

Crystal informed her that Emerald was going to be on the 6th floor if someone could take him over to see her because she was on baby duty. Alex's nurse gave him the telephone so they could speak. Crystal told him everything including the way Frank was being. "Alex?" Crystal stated. Alex replied, "Yes, what has been happening?" Crystal replied, "Frank has been arguing with everything at hospital and in the house." Alex replied, "I think it is best for him to leave the house and not return." While on the phone with Alex Frank came into the house alone. Crystal told Alex, "I love you and talk later on." Crystal let Frank be aware, "We would like you to leave the house." Frank did not agree he decided to argue he had to leave the house because Emerald needed patience and quietness to recover.

Since Alex got off the phone. Alex asked his nurse, "Can someone bring me to the 6th floor to see my daughter." Alex's nurses answered, "Let me find a volunteer that maybe available to bring you to your daughter." Alex's nurse arranged for a volunteer to take him to his baby girl who was 20 years old. He wanted to see her for himself. They went to the elevator, went up to the 6th floor while getting there Alex answered, "Can I go and see my daughter?"

The nurse at the recover desk asked, "What is your daughter's name?" Alex answered, "Her name is Emerald." The nurse looked up her name, "Please come with me." He spent half an hour while Emerald slept. She awoke briefly, saw her dad and said, "Daddy, is that you?" He reached over and felt her hand; assured her all was going to be okay. He was going to take care of everything.

Before four o'clock, Frank came storming into the house yelling. He went to grab Sapphire roughly out of Crystal's arms. Crystal said, "Hold on, Frank, settle down." He raised his arm into Crystal's face with a fist. Frank said, "That is enough, you b*t*h, get out of my face." Crystal backed up a little well saying, "enough."

Frank says, "When Emerald comes home, she will be going upstairs so will Sapphire." Crystal says, "No, neither one will be, Emerald needs time to recover totally before going upstairs to that room." Frank replied, "Like hell b*t*h she will go up if I say so." Crystal did not answer any more that Frank had to say, she already made her choice on what the next decision was being for Frank to do, as he was being very disrespectful. At that point, Joe came into the house, saw the fist in his mother's face as well as her holding the baby. He stepped between his mom and Frank. He said, "What the hell do you think you're doing Frank step away." Frank got into Joe's face yelling, "I am taking care of my family, your sister will be sleeping upstairs where she belongs no matter what this b*t*h says! She cannot stop me!"

Joe attempted to cool Frank down but realized he would not succeed, also he did not like Frank's attitude. He says, "Okay, that is my mother you are talking about! Also, she is holding onto a seven-day-old baby, so back off!" Frank wanted to fight anyone, but Joe was not going to fight him. Crystal asked Joe, "Can you take Sapphire and go upstairs with her?" Joe did just as he was asked. Crystal looked Frank eye to eye, she said what needed to be said, "Okay, Frank, this is what is going to happen: 'Doctors said her surgery was good, she is doing well, but needs time to heal.'" "Emerald does not need any undue stress, which you are causing," said Crystal.

She went on, "Also she will be weak, so no stairs." Emerald is coming home to recover, sleeping downstairs with Sapphire in her bassinet beside her. Frank started to argue, Crystal said, "That's enough; you need to get your belongings and leave now before she comes home." While he was going upstairs to get his belong, he started to yell, "You F**king B*it*h, Emerald will not agree with this," Crystal stated, "Emerald will slowly agree as she knows me, and her father only wants best for her." While Frank had his belongings and was coming down the stairs, he tried to argue but eventually left the home not to return.

After 6:00pm, Emerald was alert, the doctors came to see her. He assured her that the surgery was well, and all the afterbirth was cleared out. She needed a prescription and would be able to return home soon. She could no longer breastfeed because the toxic ions that were in her system were not good for the baby. She had concerns about Sapphire, but the doctors said, "Everything would be okay, she caught it early." He was glad at how she was looking and recovering. She was able to come home. Emerald got on the phone with Crystal, "Hey, mom, I am being discharged. Can I have someone come get me?"

Crystal let her know, "Edward will be on his way to get you." Emerald replied, "Thank you mom, see you know." Her brother Edward went to get her, he had to call the 6th floor for a volunteer to bring her to the car as he did not like hospitals.

After Emerald came home, Crystal told her all about the argument, how she and Alex decided the best thing for their daughter to recover was for Frank to leave and never come back. Emerald asks, "Mom how am I going to take care of Sapphire without someone?"

Crystal informed her, "Emerald you are a strong, independent woman who can do anything that your mind is set to do. You do not need someone like Frank bringing you done!" Emerald hugged her mom, "Mom," she whispered, "where is Sapphire." Just after Emerald asked her brother Joe walked into the living room with baby Sapphire handed her to Emerald while stating, "My amazing sister, I trust you can do anything in this world for this little bundle of joy know that you are feeling better!"

About the Author

Even though Miss Robertson became a single parent at a young age, she overcame anything that got in her way. There were financial problems as well as relationship problems. With the support of professionals, friends, and family, she was able to accomplish success. As a single parent, she would advocate for her children and their needs. She went back to school for a two-year program, which turned out to be three years. She had to be there for one of her children, but she finished the third year with a 4.0 average and a job.

www.ingramcontent.com/pod-product-compliance
Lightning Source LLC
Chambersburg PA
CBHW070037040426
42333CB00040B/1707